THE DR. SEBI

DIABETES

CURE BOOK

Shobi Nolan

Contents

CHAPTER 1

INTRODUCTION

Diabetes is a group of kidney disease that alters how the body utilizes glucose (blood sugar). Glucose is a very important substance for the body as it is the main source of energy for the body cells, even the brain cells.

Though there are different types of diabetes that have different risk factors, all diabetes usually causes excess sugar in the body. And a high level of blood sugar can lead to serious health complications.

Various types of diabetes include type 1 diabetes, type 2 diabetes, prediabetes, and gestational diabetes. Among these diabetic conditions, type 1 and type 2 diabetes are chronic and require serious medical attention, especially type 1 diabetes. Prediabetes and gestational diabetes can be easily reversed in a short period of time. Gestational diabetes usually occurs during pregnancy and reverses after delivery.

The body obtains glucose from two main sources; the liver and foods. Nonetheless, the liver releases stored glucose. Once sugar is absorbed into the bloodstream, the insulin helps it to spread throughout the entire body so that it can enter the cells. If the amount of sugar in the blood is high, some are stored in the liver as glycogen.

The stored glycogen is broken down and released as glucose when the body is in need of sugar for energy. This natural cycle helps to maintain the glucose level in the body.

CHAPTER 2

TYPE 1 DIABETES

Type 1 diabetes is an autoimmune disease that makes the immune system attack cells that produce insulin. The main causes of type 1 diabetes are yet to be confirmed. The only thing that research studies know for sure is the mechanism of type 1 diabetes. In type 1 diabetes, the immune system that protects the body against harmful microbes turns to fight against the cells that produce insulin in the pancreas.

This attack destroys the cells and renders the pancreas impotent, and thus less or no production of insulin. Consequently, the blood sugar will start to build up in the bloodstream since there is no more insulin to transport it to other cells in the body.

Risk Factors

Though the main causes of type 1 diabetes are not yet clear, it's considered to be caused by environmental factors and genetic susceptibility. Some of the factors

that may result in type 1 diabetes
are;

Family History: There is usually a
high risk of type 1 diabetes when
a member of a family or lineage
has type 1 diabetes.

Environmental Factors: Being
exposed to viral infection may
lead to type 1 diabetes. Also, the
presence of autoantibodies can
cause type 1 diabetes. However,
not everyone with autoantibodies
ends up with type 1 diabetes, but
it increases the risk.

Geography: Countries like Sweden and Finland have recorded a high rate of type 1 diabetes more than many other countries. This too can increase the risk of type 1 diabetes when other factors are put into consideration.

Other types of diabetes are gestational diabetes which usually occurs during pregnancy.

CHAPTER 4

DIABETES COMPLICATIONS

There are many health complications that can result from diabetes, especially when left untreated. These complications may be life-threatening and develop long-term. Some of these complications include;

Cardiovascular Disease:
Diabetes often results in various cardiovascular-related problems such as chest pain, stroke, heart

attack, coronary artery disease, etc.

Neuropathy: The blood vessels help to nourish your nerves. The presence of excess sugar in the bloodstream can damage the nerves if it injures the walls of the capillaries (blood vessels).

This condition often causes pain, numbness, and tingling at the tip of the fingers and toes. It may then spread to other parts of the body. If the damage reaches the digestive system, it can cause vomiting, nausea, or constipation.

Nephropathy: The tiny blood vessels in the kidney helps to remove waste from the blood. Excess sugar in the blood can damage these millions of tiny blood vessels. If damaged, it can lead to kidney failure that may require a transplant.

Retinopathy: Diabetes can lead to blindness if it damages the blood vessels in the retina. It can also cause other eye problems such as glaucoma, cataracts, etc.

CHAPTER 5

DIAGNOSIS

In most cases, the symptoms of diabetes, except type 1 diabetes, are not obvious. They are mostly neglected until the condition becomes severe. Thus, type 1 diabetes is the reason why most blood sugar tests are done. But the American Diabetes Association(ADA) has given a test guideline. This screening guidelines recommend that people under the following conditions should be tested for diabetes;

People with body mass index above 25 and with risk factors such as heart disease, high blood pressure, high cholesterol levels, polycystic ovary syndrome, sedentary lifestyle, or people with diabetic relatives.

People above 45 years of age should be screened every three years.

Women who experienced gestational diabetes should be screened every three years.

People that have had prediabetes should be screened every year.

CHAPTER 6

DR. SEBI DIET

Dr. Sebi's alkaline diet is a plant-based diet that helps to eliminate toxic wastes from the body and rejuvenate body cells.

The alkaline diet relies strictly on a list of plant foods and products approved by Dr. Sebi. Through his diet, Dr. Sebi did great wonders in people's lives; cured many diseases and revived complicated health conditions. In fact, it is one of the best plant-based diets. It was listed as one of the most popular diets in 2019.

If we can eat delicious meals and free our body from diseases, what again are we looking for? Dr. Sebi's diet can help you detox your body completely, including mucus removal, liver cleansing, diabetes reversal, cancer treatment, lupus and herpes cure, etc. Learn how to eat good foods, and you may not need medications to stay healthy.

You don't need medications to cleanse mucus from your body when you can easily get rid of it naturally by drinking and eating the right foods. By so doing, you can simply prevent and/or manage high blood pressure. The foods to take good care of your condition can be found in the nearest local grocery store.

Prepare your mind and stock your kitchen with the right foods from Dr. Sebi Approved List. Then follow the instructions in the book to help you quit smoking.

But before we get started, let's look at Dr. Sebi and his diet.

Who is Dr. Sebi?

Alfredo Darlington Bowman is an African herbalist who developed an alkaline plant diet that is based on bio-mineral balance theory. Though he is not a certified medical doctor or a Ph.D. holder, he is widely known as Dr. Sebi.

His diet is named after his popular name, The Dr. Sebi Diet. His diet was developed for those that wish to naturally detox their body for total wellness and prevent diseases by eating approved healthy plant foods.

Dr. Sebi claimed that our body is protected from diseases when it is in an alkaline state. According to him, acidic state of the body and mucus buildup in the body are the major causes of various diseases.

Though there is no scientific backup, Dr. Sebi claimed that his diet has the potential to cure lupus, sickle cell anemia, AIDS, and leukemia. He believes his diet could completely restore alkalinity in the body and detoxify the whole body.

Dr. Sebi Alkaline Diet

Dr. Sebi's diet is regarded as a vegan diet since it is a completely plant-based diet. No animal product is allowed in the diet.

Dr. Sebi claimed that this diet can make the body heal itself completely from diseases. Though there is no scientific proof for this, a lot of people who are on the diet have attested to the claim.

As a result, Dr. Sebi's diet is ranked one of the most popular diets in 2019.

The Dr. Sebi Diet Guide

Dr. Sebi's diet is solely based on plants and supplements approved by Dr. Sebi.

The diet guide can be found on his website. The simple rules to follow on Dr. Sebi diet are;

- Only foods and products listed in the nutritional guide are to be consumed.

- You must drink at least 1 gallon of water every day (that is about 3.8 liters).

- If you are on any medication, you have to take your Dr. Sebi supplements, at least, one hour before your medication.

- You don't take alcohol.

- You must not eat any animal products.

- Don't use the microwave to prepare your foods.

- Only consume naturally grown grains as listed in the guide. No wheat product is allowed.

- No seedless fruit and no canned food is permitted.

Moreover, you are expected to be using Dr. Sebi's supplements to support your diet.

CHAPTER 7

REVERSING DIABETES NATURALLY

Do you have type 2 diabetes? If you can manage to take your HbA1c below 42mmol/mol, then you have hit the jackpot. This is the aim of this book - to guide you on the road of reversing your health from a bad state to a good state. You don't need medication to do the magic. Just eat good food and live a healthy lifestyle, and you are good to go.

However, there is a need for you to consult your doctor before you make any health-related decision. Reversing diabetes seems to be a long-term process of improving your insulin sensitivity. Yes, it may be a long-term healing process. But if the body can get all the necessary tools it requires for the treatment, it can naturally surge ahead and reverse all unhealthy states in a short time.

You put diabetes in remission naturally by adhering to a life-changing diet. Coupled with other healthy lifestyles, you can make the process faster. Type 2 diabetes progression can be reversed by dropping some pounds from your body weight. If you stay dedicated to the program, the outcome is always rewarding, with full-body wellness and healing.

How Diabetes Progresses In The Body

Studies have shown that obesity is the most common risk factor for type 2 diabetes. And cutting down on the amount of weight gained through diet can be beneficial. Nevertheless, it's important we understand the mechanism through which obesity causes the progression of diabetes in the body. It seems to be a programmed cycle which must be altered to halt the progression.

When you eat foods with high amounts of refined carbohydrates and calories, it usually makes the blood insulin level increase to be able to cope with the sudden surge in carbohydrates.

As a result of the rise in insulin level, the weight starts to build up around the belly. This is known as truncal obesity. With a consistent rise in the level of insulin, the body starts to build insulin-resistant cells, which may consequently lead to weight gain.

Insulin resistance usually increases blood sugar levels after meals. The pancreas will then release more insulin that can cope with the high sugar level. This high level of insulin in the body is why you may always feel lethargic and hungry.

With a feeling of hunger, coupled with less activity, you may eat beyond what the body truly needs. This overeating, high insulin level, and inactivity will further lead to increased insulin resistance and more weight gain.

If the pancreas is overworked through high demand for insulin, the beta cells that produce the insulin may be damaged. And if damaged, the pancreas would not be able to produce enough insulin. This will result in a rise in the blood sugar level which causes diabetes.

Why You Need Dr. Sebi Diet

In order to reverse type 2 diabetes naturally, you need to follow a diet program that will cut down on the number of carbohydrates and calories you consume.

Studies have revealed that low-carb and low-calorie diets, coupled with exercise are the most effective natural means of diabetes remission.

Low-Carb Diet

A study carried out in 2014 at Naples shows that a low carbohydrate diet is very effective in reversing type 2 diabetes. According to the report, 15 percent of diabetic patients who participated in the study were able to reverse the condition after one year.

The diet is far more effective than the low-fat diet, which recorded 4 percent remission. Low carbohydrate intake is known to lower the amount of insulin required by the body.

Dr. Sebi diet is a perfect low-carb diet for you to reverse the diabetes naturally and restore good health.

Low-Calorie Diet

A low-calorie diet has relieved a lot of people from diabetes medications. It one of the effective means of weight loss and reduction of insulin resistance.

7 out of 11 diabetic patients were able to reverse their health condition after 8 weeks of

800kcal/day diet. This research at Newcastle University showed that a low-calorie diet is very active in reducing fat in the pancreas and liver.

Another study in the university on a low-calorie diet with 32 participants has recorded 40% remission so far, after 6 months of being on the diet.

However, it pertinent to note that a very-low-calorie diet is very extreme for a lot of patients. So, it's advisable to work with a certified dietitian.

Most of the approved herbs, fruits, and veggies in Dr. Sebi diet are low-calorie products that can help you reverse your health condition naturally.

Exercise

Exercise is an effective natural means of reversing type 2 diabetes as it helps the body to be more insulin sensitive. In addition to a healthy diet, it can help reverse type 2 diabetes faster.

A study carried out in 2015 recorded 67% remission after 6 months of exercise with a healthy diet.

CHAPTER 8

DR. SEBI APPROVED HERBS AND VEGETABLES

Foods with high water content and/or fiber can help the body stay hydrated, and hence prevent and cleanse excess mucus in the body. The Dr. Sebi vegetables are awesome foods with high amount of water and fiber content.

Taking these veggies will not only help you cleanse mucus, they will help your body to detox and heal naturally.

Below are some of the veggies and ways you can add them to your diet for a super healthy living.

Tomato (The Plum And Cherry)

Scientific Name: *Solanum lycopersicum*

Overview

Tomato is a popular plant grown all over the world in a temperate climate. It's widely used in different cuisines. Though it's native to western South America, China, India, the United States, and Turkey are currently the highest producers of tomatoes.

Tomato is used in many ways because of its umami flavor. It can be taken raw or cooked.

Major Compounds

Beta-carotene, lutein zeaxanthin, thiamine, niacin, vitamin B-6, vitamin C, vitamin E, vitamin K, magnesium, manganese, phosphorus, potassium

Health benefits

Heart health: Tomatoes contain high amounts of potassium and fiber. These components are important for keeping the heart healthy. Fiber helps the body to reduce cholesterol level in the blood. High consumption of potassium helps to lower the blood pressure which is good for the heart.

Healthy bone: Phosphorus, magnesium, and vitamin C play crucial roles in the development of string and healthy bones. Tomatoes contain high amounts of phosphorus and moderate amounts of magnesium and vitamin C.

Eye health: The lutein and beta-carotene found in tomatoes are needed by our eyes to protect the retina and keep the eye free from macular degeneration.

Prevents cancer: tomatoes contain several vitamins and antioxidants such as lycopene, beta-carotene, vitamin C, etc. These components have properties that enables them to fight cancer cells and free radicals that can cause damage to the body cells.

How To Use

Tomatoes are used in many ways. It can be eaten raw or cooks. It can be used to make side dishes. Awesome for fruit and vegetable salads. Tomorrow is the major ingredient for stew. Many use it to cook soup, make sandwiches, or add it to wraps.

There are so many ways to use it. It can be used for smoothies and juice.

Nutrition fact

Per 100g

- Calories: 18 kcal
- Carbs: 3.9g
- Sugars: 2.6g
- Fiber: 1.2g
- Fat: 0.2g
- Protein: 0.9g

Side Effects

Excessive intake of tomatoes can lead to some unhealthy conditions. Some of these side effects include diarrhea, acid reflux, headache, kidney stones, lycopenodermia, joint pain, severe throat/mouth irritation, vomiting, mild spasms, dizziness, etc.

Squash

Scientific Name: *Cucurbita spp.*

Overview

Squash is a widely used food crop that originated from Mexico. Now popular in the South, North America, and Asia. India and China have been the highest producers of squash so far.

There are different types of squashes with several color variations. Squash has fed many mouths and is still feeding a lot at the moment. It is cooked and used in different dishes.

Major Compounds

Beta-carotene, lutein, zeaxanthin, thiamine, riboflavin, niacin, pantothenic acid, vitamin B6, folate, vitamin C, vitamin K, iron, magnesium, manganese, phosphorus, potassium, zinc, oleic, palmitic, and linoleic fatty acids.

Health benefits

Heart health: Fiber and potassium are important substances that help to take care of the heart. High fiber content foods help to reduce the cholesterol level in our blood.

Enough intake of potassium helps the body to lower blood pressure. Squash contains a high amount of potassium which is vital to the heart.

Cancer: squash contains important antioxidants that may help the body to prevent cancer. Some of these antioxidants reduce the growth rate of cancer cells and help to protect the body cells against free radicals.

Healthy Eye: Squash contains beta-carotene and lutein, which are important compounds for healthy eyes. They help to protect the retina and keep the eyes free from macular degeneration.

How To Use

Simply wash and peel off the skin. Then use as you desire. You can cook your squash, or roast it. Smashed and used as an ingredient for other dishes like soup.

Some squash have tough cover. To peel them off you need to put them in your oven for about 2 minutes, with the skin pierced with a fork. Or bake/cook with the skin on. Then it will be easier to remove the skin.

Nutrition fact

Per 100g

- Calories: 16 kcal

- Carbs: 3.4g

- Sugars: 2.2g

- Fiber: 1.1g

- Fat: 0.2g

- Protein: 1.2g

Side Effects

Some of the side effects associated with the use of squash

include allergic reactions such as dermatitis, itching, difficulty in breathing, nasal congestion, swelling of face and lips, etc.

Onion

Scientific Name*: Allium cepa*

Overview

Onion is one of the most popular food ingredients used worldwide. Though its origin has many claims, the only fact is that onion originated from Asia.

It is widely cultivated all over the world. It can be eaten raw or cooked. Onion can be pungent to the eye when exposed. Three types of onions are predominant; the yellow onion, red onion, and white onion. All

are flavorful and super healthy
for use.

Major Compounds
Polyphenols, thiamine, riboflavin,
niacin, pantothenic acid, vitamin
B-6, folate, vitamin C, calcium,
iron, magnesium, manganese,
phosphorus, potassium, zinc

Health benefits
Cancer: the antioxidants in
onions can help the body to fight
against cancer by protecting the
body cells against oxidative
damage. They can reduce the

growth of cancer cells, and thus, helps to reduce the risk of cancer.

Heart health: fiber in our foods helps to lower the level of cholesterol in our body. Moreover, the high amount of potassium in onions plays a vital role in the reduction of blood pressure. These properties of onions plus more ensure a healthy heart.

Osteoporosis: Calcium, potassium, and vitamin C are important to the bone. These compounds provided in good amounts by onion can help the body to develop strong and healthy bones.

Anti-inflammatory: Destroying radical cells that are toxic to the body is one of the means our body uses to prevent inflammation. The antioxidants from onions help the body to fight against these radicals.

How To Use

Onion is used to prepare most dishes.

First peel off the outer layer and wash. Dice or slice to your taste and add to your food; salads, wraps, sandwiches, soup, stew, etc. It can be taken raw or cooked. Anyway, it is super healthy for consumption.

Nutrition fact

Per 100g

- Calories: 40

- Fat: 0.1g

- Carbs: 9g

- Fiber: 1.7g

- Sugar: 4.2g

- Protein: 1.1g

Side Effects

Some of the side effects
associated with the use of onions
include blurred vision, dermatitis,
bronchial asthma, itching,
sweating, and anaphylaxis

Olive

Scientific Name: *Olea europaea*

Overview

Dominant in the Mediterranean region, olive is a very important ingredient in the Mediterranean foods. It has wonderful health benefits. Some people claim that it is the healthiest food on earth and one of the oldest known trees, thanks to its religious attachment.

Though olive is not native to the Americas, it is one of the most popular ingredients used in America, especially the oil.

Major Compounds

potassium, calcium, magnesium, vitamin E, phosphorus, sodium, polyphenol, iron, choline

Health benefits

Heart health: olive contains carbohydrates that are mostly made up of fiber. This high fiber content of olive helps the body to lower cholesterol levels.

Diabetes: research suggests that food with high fiber content strongly helps to reduce blood sugar levels. Olive is a good source of fiber and consuming a good amount of olive will help prevent and possibly treat type 2 diabetes.

Anti-inflammatory: olive contains wonderful compounds and antioxidants that help to protect the body cells against oxidative damages, which may lead to inflammation of the body.

Cancer: the antioxidants provided by olive helps to reduce the growth of cancer cells in the body. Thus, taking olive can help one to prevent cancer cell formation.

How To Use

Olive is cultivated for different use. But most people cultivate olive for its oil which is the most used oil in the Mediterranean diet.

Nutrition fact

Per 100 g

- Calories: 146 kcal

- Carbs: 3.84g

- Sugars: 0.54g

- Fiber: 3.3g

- Fat: 15.32g

- Protein: 1.03g

Side Effects

There is no enough record on the side effects of olive. But there could be possible allergic reactions. If you have a complicated health condition, consult your physician before use.

Okra

Scientific Name: *Abelmoschus esculentus*

Overview

Okra is a widely used vegetable all over the world. Some regions call it Okro or ladies' finger. This healthy plant that originated from West Africa has a mucilaginous property. This makes most foods cooked with okra to be slimy, unless it's deslimed. One of the things mostly used to deslime okra is tomato.

This healthy vegetable is widely cultivated for food because of its nutritional values. It is used in many ways such as in making salads, soups, stews, etc.

Major Compounds

Protein, carbohydrates, fiber, vitamin K, vitamin C, thiamin, folate, magnesium, riboflavin, niacin, potassium, calcium, iron, phosphorus, zinc, flavonoids, and isoquercetin

Health benefits

Prevention of Cancer: okra contains lectin and folate. Researches suggest that these compounds strongly inhibit the growth of cancer cells. Thus, taking enough okra can help one to prevent the risk of cancer.

Pregnancy: The folate gotten from okra helps to keep a healthy pregnancy. Lack of folate in the body may possibly lead to miscarriage.

Prevents diabetes: Test done on animals (rat) shows that okra can reduce the fat and blood sugar level in the body.

Heart health: Okra provides the body with useful fibers which can help to keep the heart-healthy. American Heart Association (AHA) suggests that food with high fiber content helps the body to reduce cholesterol level.

Osteoporosis: okra provides a high amount of calcium and vitamin K to the body. Calcium and vitamin K are very vital for the development of strong and healthy bones.

How To Use

Okra can be used in many ways. It can be taken raw, roasted, pickled, fried, boiled, or sauteed. You can add it to your soup, salads, or other foods.

To remove the sliminess of okra in your food, try and cook it over high heat and avoid cooking in a crowded pot. You can also pickle it or cook with acidic food like tomato.

Nutrition fact

Per 100g

- Calories: 33

- Fat: 0.2g

- Carbs: 7g

- Fiber: 3.2g

- Sugar: 1.5g

- Protein: 1.9g

Side Effects

Some side effects associated with the use of okra include cramping, diarrhea, gas, and bloating.

Nopals

Scientific Name*: Opuntia spp.*

Overview

Native to Mexico, nopales is a food ingredient with important health benefits. There are about 114 species of nopales in Mexico. This highly medicinal food is not popular like other herbs such as lettuces, kale, etc, but it is common among the residents of southwest America.

It's popularly known in English as "prickly pear".

Major Compounds

Manganese, vitamin C, magnesium, calcium, antioxidants, sodium, potassium

Health benefits

Antiviral: research suggests that nopales gas antiviral properties that can be used against herpes and HIV.

Antioxidant: Nopales have a high content of antioxidants which help to protect the body cells against radical damage and reduce oxidative stress.

Blood Sugar Level: research has it that nopales have important properties that can help to regulate blood sugar levels.

Cholesterol: earlier studies suggest that nopales can lower cholesterol levels, especially LDL cholesterol.

Enlarged Prostate: Nopales may help to reduce enlarged prostate, which is a serious health condition for men. It may as well help to treat prostate cancer.

How To Use

Nopales can be eaten raw or cooked. It can be used to make juice, jams, smoothies, tea, etc.

It can be prepared with other Dr. Sebi approved foods as side dishes, salads, etc.

Nutrition fact
Per 100g

- Calories: 16

- Total Fat: 0.1g

- Fiber: 2g

- Sugar: 1.1g

- Protein: 1.4g

Side Effects

Some of the side effects associated with nopales include bloating, headache, diarrhea, nausea

Mushrooms

Scientific Name: *Agaricus bisporus*

Overview

With over 14,000 types, mushrooms are widely cultivated all over the world for commercial and medicinal use. China, Italy, and the United States are known to be among the highest producers of mushrooms.

The most consumed mushroom until this century remains the white mushrooms. There are many health benefits associated with mushrooms and that is one of the major reasons why it gained its popularity.

However, not all mushrooms are edible as some can be highly toxic to the body. There are over 2,000 edible mushrooms. Among the edible ones shiitake is not approved for the Dr Sebi diet. So, it's pertinent that one should avoid shitake and any other mushroom that is not edible.

Major Compounds

Protein, pantothenic acid, riboflavin, niacin, copper, calcium, selenium, potassium, fiber, vitamin D, ergothioneine, glutathione

Health benefits

Cancer Prevention: The antioxidants in mushrooms can help to prevent cancer cells from reproducing. Thus, mushrooms help the body to lower the risk of cancer.

Neurodegenerative Disease (Alzheimer's): Ergothioneine and glutathione which are majorly produced by mushrooms are claimed to be potentially useful for the treatment of

Alzheimer's and Parkinson's diseases

Heart Health: Mushrooms are one of the major producers of potassium. High intake of potassium helps to reduce blood pressure.

Diabetes: The fiber content of mushrooms can help to fight against diabetes. Fiber is known to be useful in managing type 2 diabetes.

How To Use

First trim the end of the stalk, clean, and wash before use. It can be sliced, diced, or used the whole. Though it can be taken raw, cooked mushrooms are most preferred.

Mushrooms can be used to make salads, side dishes, pizza, scrambles, quiche, omelette, sandwiches, wraps, etc.

Nutrition fact

Per 100g

- Calories: 22

- Fat: 0.3g

- Total Carbs: 3.3g

- Fiber: 1g

- Sugar: 2g

- Protein: 3.1g

Side Effects

Dryness of the mouth or throat, rashes, diarrhea, itchiness, stomach upset, cramps, headache, nausea, vomiting, and diarrhea

Dandelion

Scientific Name: *Taraxacum officinale*

Overview

Dandelion is a herbaceous plant grown all over the world for food and medicinal purposes. It's claimed to have a myriad of medicinal properties that can be used in the prevention and potential cure for physical ailments.

Native to North America and Eurasia, dandelion is widely consumed as a nutritious food. All parts of the plant are edible, including the flower, leaves, roots, and stems.

The flowers are known to contain high amounts of phytochemicals, with the leaves rich in lutein, while the root has a lot of probiotic fibers.

Major Compounds

Vitamin A, folate, vitamin K, vitamin C, calcium, potassium, iron, manganese, polyphenols, inulin, lutein, beta-carotene

Health benefits
Good Source of Antioxidants:
dandelion provides the body with

a good amount of antioxidants such as beta-carotene and polyphenols which help to protect the body cells against radical damages.

Regulation of Cholesterol Levels: researches done on animals suggests that dandelion is very effective in reducing cholesterol levels. It also lowers the amount of fat in the liver, which means that dandelion can be used for the treatment of fatty liver disease.

Blood Sugar Regulation: the antihyperglycemic, anti-inflammatory and antioxidative properties found in dandelion can be useful for the treatment of type 2 diabetes.

Anti-inflammatory: chemical extracts from dandelion are claimed to be potent in the reduction of body inflammation.

Blood Pressure Regulation: potassium is known to be an effective supplement for lowering blood pressure.

Weight Loss: the chlorogenic acid found in dandelion can be effective in reducing weight and lipid accumulation.

Prevention of Cancer: Research suggests that dandelion can be highly effective in the prevention of cancer as it has the potential to inhibit the growth of cancer cells.

Immune System Boost: The antibacterial and antiviral properties of dandelion can be useful for the immune system. Research suggests that dandelion can inhibit the growth of hepatitis B.

How To Use

Dandelion can be used in many ways. Depending on how you want it, it's mostly preferred when blanched to remove some bitterness. It can be taken raw (both fresh and dried), added to smoothies, teas, and juice, or used to make salads. It can be added to soup. The root can be roasted and used as coffee.

Nutrition fact

Per 100g

- Calories: 45

- Total Fat: 0.7g

- Total Carbs: 9.2g

- Fiber: 3.5g

- Sugar: 0.7g

- Protein: 2.7g

Side Effects

There is no enough record on the side effect on the use of dandelions. But dandelion can cause allergic reactions, diarrhea, or heartburn.

Lettuce

Scientific Name: Lactuca sativa

Overview

Lettuce which originated from Egypt and mostly produced in China is widely known for its wonderful health benefits. Some people call it the perfect weight-loss food.

It can be used in diverse ways for various purposes, especially for medicinal purposes. In many regions, it is used for the treatment of typhoid, body pain, smallpox, rheumatism, coughs, and nervousness - even insanity, though there is no scientific backup for this claim.

There are different types of lettuce which include leaf lettuce, romaine lettuce, iceberg, summercrip, butterhead, red leaf, oilseed, and celtuce.

Note: Iceberg is not approved by Dr. Sebi.

Major Compounds

Vitamin K, vitamin A (beta-carotene, lutein, zeaxanthin), folate, iron, thiamine, riboflavin, pantothenic acid, vitamin c, vitamin e, calcium, magnesium,

manganese, phosphorus,
potassium, sodium, zinc

Health benefits

Prevents Dehydration: lettuce,
especially red lettuce is made up
of 96% water. This can help to
keep the body hydrated.

Antioxidant: lettuce contains a
lot of antioxidants such as beta-
carotene which helps to protect
the body cells against radical
damage. Antioxidants play vital
roles in the wholesome wellness
of our bodies.

Heart Health: the presence of potassium in lettuce may help to lower the level of blood pressure.

Eye Health: The beta-carotene and other antioxidants got from lettuce help to protect the eye from macular degeneration.

Prevents Diabetes: Lettuce has a low glycemic index and zero glycemic loads which are good for those trying to lower their blood sugar, especially for managing type 2 diabetes.

How To Use

First wash the lettuce, pound on a chopping board to make it soft. Separate the leaves and dry. Then tear into smaller parts and dress.

Lettuce can be used to make smoothies, salads, and sandwiches. It can also be added to soups and wraps.

Nutrition fact

Per 100g

- Calories: 15

- Fat: 0.2g

- Carbs: 2.9g

- Fiber: 1.3g

- Sugar: 0.8g

- Protein: 1.4g

Side Effects

Some of the potential side effects associated with lettuce consumption include sweating, itching, fast heartbeat, nausea, vomiting, pupil dilation, diarrhea, dizziness, ringing in the ears, vision rashes, vision changes, sedation, and breathing difficulty.

Izote

Scientific Name: *Yucca gigantea*

Overview

Commonly known as yucca, izote is a garden plant that is native to Central America and Mexico. It is claimed to have varieties of medicinal properties. It is one of the most popular sources of saponin, a natural detergent.

Generally, it is cultivated as a houseplant, ornamental garden, herb, or food. Thus, it is used in diverse ways, especially in the treatment of illness like arthritis.

Though it can survive in different soils and conditions, it thrives most in hot semi-arid or warm climates.

Health benefits

Arthritis: According to research, the chemical extracts from izotes can potentially help in the treatment of arthritis.

Heart Health: steroidal saponins from izote helps the body to lower cholesterol level in the blood. This helps to keep the heart healthy.

Prevention of Cancer: the phenols gotten from izote can help to prevent the growth of cancer cells, and thus, eliminating any potential risk of cancer.

Anti-inflammatory: izote contains phenols like resveratrol and yuccaols A, B, C, D and E, which are known to be anti-inflammatory.

How To Use

First remove the ovaries and anthers. Then blanch for about 5 minutes. You can cook your izote

with onion, tomatoes, and chile.
Bool and eat with lemon juice, or
use it with egg-battered patties.

Side Effects

Some possible side effects
associated with izote are upset
stomach, bitter taste, vomiting,
nausea.

Kale

Scientific Name: *Brassica oleracea*

Overview

Kale is one of the most popular veggies in the world. It is highly nutritious and heavily used for its medicinal properties.

It's claimed to originate from Asia Minor and Eastern Mediterranean where it was cultivated for food. Kale is best cultivated in the winter times for maximum yield.

Major Compounds

Protein, fiber, vitamins A, C, and K, folate, alpha-linolenic acid, lutein and zeaxanthin, phosphorus, potassium, calcium, zinc, carotenoids, phenols

Health benefits

Diabetes: The fiber content of kale can play an important role in the prevention and treatment of diabetes since fiber helps to regulate blood sugar level.

Antioxidants: kale contains a high amount of antioxidants

which help to protect the body cells against oxidative damage.

Heart health: high intake of potassium and reduction in the consumption of sodium helps to lower the risk of high blood pressure. Moreover, fiber in our diet helps to lower cholesterol level. These properties help to take care of the heart.

Prevention Cancer: The presence of antioxidants in our body helps to protect our cells and hinder the development of cancer cells.

Healthy Eye: the lutein and zeaxanthin gotten from kale help to protect our eyes against macular degeneration. Vitamins, zinc, and beta-carotene help to protect the retina and keep the eyes healthy.

Healthy Bone: Calcium and vitamin K are very important for the development of healthy bones. Even, phosphorus and vitamin D also support the health of our bones.

Healthy skin and Hair: the human skin needs beta-carotene and vitamin A for development and maintenance of body tissues. Also, the vitamin C provided by kale helps to build and support the protein, collagen, responsible for skin and hair growth

How To Use

You can use kale in many ways. Kale can be eaten raw, steamed, or sauteed. Gently scrunch the kale leaf to make it soft. Then add it to your salads, sandwiches, and smoothies, wraps. Blend with other veggies and fruits to make smoothies and juice. Saute with onion for a side dish. You can spice it up and bake for 15-30 minutes to make your kale chips.

Nutrition fact

Per 100g

- Calories: 49

- Fat: 0.9g

- Total Carbs: 9g

- Protein: 4.3g

Side Effects

If you are battling with hypothyroidism, kale is not the best vegetable for you. Consult

your physician for your diets.
Excessive intake of kale can
inhibit the production of thyroid
hormone.

Garbanzo Beans

Scientific Name: *Cicer arietinum*

Overview

Garbanzo beans is a nutrient-dense legume which is highly cultivated almost in all parts of the world. It is highly rich in fiber, protein, folate, iron, etc.

There are two types of garbanzo, the big size with light color, which ich predominant in the Americas and the small size with dark color that is mainly found in the Middle East and India

However, American garbanzo beans are far sweeter than the Indian garbanzo beans. This is one of those foods that takes time to cook, but it always comes out with great taste.

Major Compounds

Protein, folate, fiber, iron, phosphorus, fatty acids, sitosterol,

Health benefits

Diabetes: Beans are known to be slow in digestion. Garbanzo beans have a very low glycerin index (GI) and glycemic load (GL).

These properties help to reduce blood sugar and insulin levels. Thus, it can be used to control the sugar level of patients with type 2 diabetes.

Heart Disease: the plant sterol in garbanzo beans known as sitosterol helps to lower the cholesterol level in the blood.

Obesity: the high fiber content of garbanzo beans can help to promote weight loss. High fiber content in a diet makes one have the feeling of fullness, and this satiating effect helps in weight loss.

How To Use

First sort the beans to remove stones and debris. Then soak overnight and cook for about 1 or 2 hours, depending on the heat you are using. Check for recipes and get directions. You can use the cooked garbanzo beans in many ways.

It can be added to your stew, soup, or salad. You can make hummus with it by blending it with olive oil, lemon juice, garlic, and tahini. Mashed and used in place of flour.

Roast and grind to make coffee.

Nutrition fact

Per 100g

- Calories: 378 kcal
- Carbs: 62.95g
- Sugars: 10.7g
- Fiber: 12.2g
- Fats: 6.04g
- Protein: 20.47g

Side Effects

Some of the side effects recorded on the use of garbanzo beans include stomach cramp, gas pains, and discomfort. The allergies associated include redness, rashes, inflammation, diarrhea, and hives.

Cucumber

Scientific Name: *Cucumis sativus*

Overview

Cucumber is a creeping vine plant that is cultivated all over the world. According to history, cucumbers originated form India before spreading to other parts of the world.

It contains about 95% water which makes it one of the best fruits/vegetables to manage dehydration. It is cultivated for both food and medicinal purposes as it contains healthy substances that are highly beneficial to the body.

Major Compounds

Calcium, potassium, magnesium, phosphorus, iron, sodium, vitamin C, beta-carotene, folate, lutein zeaxanthin, nantothenic acid, cucurbitacin, vitamin K, vitamin B-6, thiamine, riboflavin, niacin

Health benefits

Hydration: hydration is one of the major benefits of cucumber as it is made up of 95% water. This water is super healthy as it has important electrolytes which helps to prevent constipation and maintain healthy intestine.

Healthy Bone: vitamin and calcium are very important for the bone. Calcium keeps the bone strong and healthy while vitamin K facilitate the absorption of calcium. Also, vitamin D supports the heath if the bone.

Cancer Prevention:
Cucurbitacin is a nutrient know to inhibit cancer cells from reproducing and hence prevents the development of cancer cells.

Heart Health: The fiber content of cucumber helps to regulate cholesterol levels and prevent possible heart disease.

Diabetes Prevention: Cucumber has low glycerin index, which means it has low potential of increasing blood sugar. Also, according to American Heart Association (AHA), fiber helps to prevent type 2 diabetes.

How To Use

Cucumber is usually eaten raw. You can add it to your salads or sandwiches. Use it to make side dishes and have a good meal time. For your smoothies and juice, you can blend cucumber and add it.

There is no specific limitation to the use of cucumber. You can add it to any food you feel like enjoying with cucumber. The most important thing is for it to add value to your health and also give you a great taste.

Nutrition Facts

Per 100g

- Calories: 65 kJ (16 kcal)

- Carbs: 3.63g

- Sugars: 1.67

- Dietary fiber: 0.5 g

- Fat: 0.11 g

- Protein: 0.65 g

Side Effects

Excessive amount of vitamin K may affect blood clotting. So it's advisable to consume reasonable amount of cucumber since it contains a lot vitamin K.

Some allergies associated with the consumption of cucumber include swelling and hives. Some people also report of difficult breathing. So, watch out for thethese signs.

Chayote

Scientific Name*: Sechium edule*

Overview

Chayote originated from Mexico and many parts of Latin America. Now it's grown all over the world. It's also known as choko or mirliton. It is mainly used when cooked.

Almost all part of this pear-shaped plant is edible, including the root, leaves, stem, and seeds. It contains loads of nutrients that can help transform and keep the body healthy.

Major Compounds

Potassium, vitamin C, magnesium, folate, manganese, vitamin K, vitamin B-6, zinc, quercetin, myricetin, morin, kaem pferol

Health benefits
Promotes Heart Health:

according to researchers, some chayote compounds help to reduce blood pressure and improve blood flow.

Also, Myricetin which is provided by the body helps to reduce the level of cholesterol in the body.

Moreover, taking fiber-rich foods helps to lower the risk of heart disease - chayote is one of the fiber-rich foods.

Blood Sugar Control: the fiber content of chayote helps to promote insulin sensitivity and regulation of blood sugar.

Support Healthy Pregnancy: The folate provided by chayote helps to lower the risk of miscarriage during pregnancy.

Anticancer: the myricetin in chayote has a strong anticancer property which helps to fight against cancer.

Anti-Aging: Chayote is loaded with a high amount of antioxidants which help to protect the body cells against oxidative damage. Also, since vitamin C is verily vital in the production of collagen, the high amount of vitamin C in chayote ensures the skin stays firm and youthful.

Prevents Liver Disease:
Excessive deposits of fats in the

liver leads to fatty liver disease. Test tube and animal studies suggest that chayote extract can help to protect the liver by preventing the accumulation of fats in the liver.

Support Digestion: The fiber and flavonoids from chayote keep the digestive tract healthy as they keep the digestive enzymes in the gut healthy and remove wastes from the digestive tract, respectively.

How To Use

Chayote is mainly used when cooked, roasted, steamed, or fried. You can also eat it raw by adding it to your salads and smoothies.

You can add it to stews, soups, casserole dishes.

Nutrition fact

Per 100g

- Calories: 19
- Fat: 0.1g
- Cholesterol: 0mg
- Sodium: 2mg
- Potassium: 125mg

- Carbs: 4.5g

- Fiber: 1.7g

- Sugar: 1.7 g

- Protein: 0.8 g

Side Effects

Allergic reactions

Bell Pepper

Scientific Name: *Capsicum annuum*

Overview

Bell peppers are 5% carbs and 94% water, with minute protein and fats.

Native to Central America, Mexico, and South America, it is cultivated in warm climate and moist soil of about 70 - 84F temperature.

It does not burn strongly like other peppers because it does not produce lipophilic chemical, capsaicin, that is responsible for the burning sensation from peppers.

Bell peppers have different colors including orange, yellow, red, and green (when unripe).

Major Compounds

Potassium, vitamins c, b-6, e, a, and k1, folate, capsanthin, violaxanthin, lutein, quercetin, luteolin,

Health benefits

Eye Health: the carotenoids, lutein and zeaxanthin, provided in large amounts by bell peppers protect the retina from oxidative damage.

Prevention Of Anemia: Iron deficiency is the major cause of weakness and tiredness of the body which is a result of the blood not being able to carry enough oxygen.

The vitamin C provided by the bell pepper promotes the absorption of iron into the body system.

How To Use

Bell pepper can be eaten raw or
cooked. You can use your bell
pepper in garden salads. It can
be used as toppings on your
cheese steaks and pizza. You can
use it for your stuffed peppers.
You can dry and powder it to
make paprika spice.

Nutrition fact

Per 100g

- Calories: 31

- Water: 92%

- Protein: 1g

- Carbs: 6g

- Sugar: 4.2g

- Fiber: 2.1g

- Fat: 0.3g

Side Effects

Nausea, loose stools, mild burning sensation, sneezing, stomach pain, watery eyes

Arugula

Scientific Name: *Eruca vesicaria*

Overview

Native to the Mediterraneans, arugula is a leafy green vegetable with fresh, bitter, tart, and peppery-mustard flavor. It is popularly known is some regions as garden rocket, roquette, rucola, or colewort. It is widely used as healthy ingredient for salads.

It is super nutrition and may help the body to prevent the risk of cancer, eye damage, or osteoporosis and arthritis.

Major Compounds

Potassium, calcium, phosphorus, vitamin k, vitamin b-6, vitamin c, magnesium, sodium, thiamine, riboflavin, dietary fiber, fat, protein, vitamin a, beta-carotene, lutein zeaxanthin, niacin, vitamin e, iron,

Health Benefits

Healthy Bone: Calcium, vitamin K, magnesium, and phosphorus supplied by arugula are the major minerals for the development of strong and healthy bone. These minerals helps the body to prevent any risk of osteoporosis and arthritis.

Heart Health: Arugula contains wonderful minerals to take care of the body naturally. Arugula contains high amount of potassium, vitamins and antioxidants, with moderate amount of fiber which help to protect the heart. The fiber helps the body to lower and regulate the level of cholesterol in the blood, while the potassium reduces blood pressure.

Cancer: The vitamins and antioxidants from arugula help the body to prevent the formation of cancer cells. They also protect the body cells against radical damage. This also aids anti-inflammation.

Eye Health: The high content of vitamin A, lutein and b-carotene in arugula protect and help the eyes to fight against macular degeneration.

How To Use

First rinse with cold water and dry. In addition to the leaves and seeds, it is good to know that the young seed pods, and flowers of arugula are also edible. They can be used to make salads. It can be added to soups, or used to make sauce. Some people also use it for their pizza.

Side Effects

Some possible side effects with excessive consumption of arugula include abdominal cramping, flatulence, and discomfort.

Turnip Greens

Scientific Name: *Brassica rapa var. rapa*

Overview

Turnip greens are root vegetables widely cultivated worldwide as food crop. It thrives better in the temperate climates. Turnip green is known as one of the best sources of vitamins and regarded as one of the healthiest vegetables in the world.

During winter and late autumn, turnip is the most common side dish in southeastern region of United

States. It's fully packed with antioxidants, potassium, calcium, and fiber.

Major Compounds

potassium, phosphorus, magnesium, vitamin K, folate, vitamin C, zinc, iron, sodium, Lutein, beta-Carotene,

Health Benefits

Heart Health: Turnip contains wonderful substances to take care of the body naturally. Turnip contains high amount of potassium, fiber, vitamins and antioxidants which help to protect the heart. The fiber helps the body to lower and regulate the level of cholesterol in the blood, while the potassium is a good mineral used by the body to reduce blood pressure.

Hair and Skin Care: Vitamin C in one of the major vitamins supplied by turnip to the body. Vitamin C helps the body to build and maintain collagen. Vitamin A is vital for all body tissues including those for skin and hair. While iron helps to stop hair loss.

Healthy Bone: Calcium, vitamin K, vitamin D, magnesium, and phosphorus supplied by turnip are the major minerals for the development of strong and healthy bone. These minerals helps the body to prevent any risk of osteoporosis.

Pregnancy Care: The vitamins and minerals produced by turnip are vital to keep a healthy pregnancy. Folate in the body protects pregnant women from the risk of miscarriage.

Cancer: The vitamins and antioxidants from turnip helps the to prevent the development of cancer cells. They also protect the body cells against free radical which could cause serious damage to body cells. This also aids anti-inflammation.

Eye Health: The high content of lutein and b-carotene protects and helps fight against macular degeneration.

Diabetes: Fiber is known to help in managing type 2 diabetes as it helps to regulate blood sugar.

How To Use

First rinse with cold water, and slice as desired. Turnip can be eaten raw or cooked. You can add turnip to your salad or smoothie. It can be sauteed or boiled, and added to soups, casserole, or other dishes. Side dish for rice and beans,

Side Effects

Though turnip is a wonderful source of healthy minerals, too much consumption of it may not be healthy for the body since it contains high amount of these minerals already.

Some of the possible side effects that could be associated with the consumption of turnip include runny nose, cough, watery eyes, lip swelling and redness, sore eyes, sinus, breathing problems, etc.

Watercress

Scientific Name: *Nasturtium officinale*

Overview

Watercress is a rapid growing flowering plant that is widely used in Europe and Asia. It is native to these two continents, but has found its wide use in other regions like the Americas. It is known to be one of the oldest vegetables on earth.

It is an aquatic plant and thus, perfect for hydroponic cultivation. It is used in different delicacies and it is highly nutritious. It can be eaten raw or cooked.

Major Compounds

potassium, calcium, vitamin K, phosphorus, folate, magnesium, vitamin C, vitamin A, beta-Carotene, lutein zeaxanthin, vitamin E, riboflavin, vitamin B-6, manganese, thiamine, pantothenic acid, iron, sodium

Health Benefits

Heart Health: Watercress contains high amount of potassium, vitamins and antioxidants which may help to keep a healthy heart. High amount of potassium helps the body to reduce blood pressure.

Skin Care: Vitamin C helps the body to build and maintain collagen while vitamin A is vital for tissue development including those for skin.

Healthy Bone: Calcium, vitamin K, vitamin C, and phosphorus from watercress are essential minerals in the formation of strong and healthy bone. These minerals keeps the bones free from osteoporosis and arthritis.

Cancer: The vitamins and antioxidants from turnip helps to prevent the build up of cancer cells. They also protect the body cells against oxidative damage to body cells.

Eye Health: The amount of lutein and b-carotene in watercress is very high and they can help to protect the eye from macular degeneration.

Other Possible Health Benefits

Some people use watercress as a short-term solution for inflammation of the lungs, baldness, and sexual arousal.

How To Use

Mostly used to make salads, watercress can be used in other foods like soup, omelet, scrambled egg, pasta sauce. It can be added to sandwiches, wraps, smoothies, and juice.

Side Effects

There is no enough record on the possible side effects of watercress. It is advisable to use moderate amount of watercress, and then watch out for any possible side effects.

Purslane

Scientific Name: *Portulaca oleracea*

Overview

Purslane is a leafy green vegetable with sour and salty taste. Wide known as weed because of its ability to survive in harsh conditions, unlike other green veggies. It is more common as edible vegetable in the Middle East, Europe, and Asia. Even the Mexicans are used to it.

It can be eaten raw as salad or used in several delicacies. Its

mucilaginous property makes it
perfect for soups and stews.

Major Compounds

potassium, calcium, magnesium,
phosphorus, folate, vitamin B-6,
vitamin E, vitamin C, vitamin A,
iron, manganese, thiamine, niacin,
riboflavin, zinc

Health Benefits

Anti-inflammatory: The
vitamins gotten from purslane
have anti-inflammatory and
antioxidant properties. These
properties help to protect body
cells against free radicals and

thus, keep the body free from inflammation. It may also be essential for cancer prevention.

Heart Health: Purslane is one of the best sources of potassium among leafy greens. Thus, may be essential for the heart, since potassium helps to reduce blood pressure.

Skin Care: Vitamin C and E the major vitamins supplied by purslane to the body. Vitamin C is known to be vital for collagen while vitamin E plays a vital role in cell regeneration. These vitamins help to keep the skin free from blemishes.

Healthy Bone: Calcium, magnesium and phosphorus provided by purslane are essential minerals for strong and healthy bones. These minerals help to to prevent and treat osteoporosis and arthritis.

How To Use

Purslane's leaves, stems, and flower buds are very much edible and they are highly nutritious. Purslane can be used in salads and soups. It is good for stir-fries.

It is good to know that the fresh young leaves are the best for use.

Some people apply fresh purslane leaf on the skin to treat burns, and other skin ailments.

Side Effects

Enough data have not been recorded on the side effects associated with the use purslane.

Amaranth Greens

Scientific Name: *Amaranthus dubious*

Overview

Amaranth Greens are herbaceous edible leafy vegetables that are native to Mexico and Central America. In the pre-Columbian time, it is one of the healthiest staple foods cultivated by the Aztecs and Incas.

Nowadays, it's mostly cultivated in the tropical climate of Asia, Latin America, and Africa where it flowers from some to fall.

In the subtropical environment, it can flower throughout the year.

In India, China, and Africa amaranth is usually cultivated as leafy-vegetable. The Europeans and Americans cultivate amaranth for their grains.

Health Benefits

- The stems and leaves contain a healthy amount of insoluble and soluble dietary fiber. This is why it is highly recommended by dieticians for a weight loss program and control of cholesterol levels in the body.

- Amaranth leaves are known to contain no zero cholesterol and a good amount of healthy fats. The greens contain approximately 23 calories/100g.

- Amaranth greens are vital for complete wellness of the body as they contain adequate amounts of antioxidants, vitamins, phytonutrients, and minerals required by the body.

- Iron is one of the essential components for the production of red blood cells. During cellular metabolism, iron serves as a co-factor for cytochrome oxidase (oxidation-reduction enzyme). A fresh Amaranth green of about 100g carries 29% DRI of iron.

- Amaranth greens contain a high amount of potassium, even more than spinach. Potassium is a very important mineral in the cells and body fluids. It helps to regulate blood pressure and heart rate.

- It also contains high amounts of magnesium, calcium, manganese, zinc, and copper, which are vital components for the body cells.

- Like other greens, amaranth helps the body in preventing weakness of the bone, which is known as iron-deficiency anemia (osteoporosis).

How To Use
For the grain:

- Add to water twice the volume of the grain or 2.4 times the weight of the grain and boil.

For the leave:

- Separate the leaf and stem.

- Wash the leaf with cold water and gently pat dry with a tissue.

- Then chop before you use it in any recipe. It can also be used without chopping.

- Do not overcook the amaranth leaf so you don't destroy most of its nutrients, especially the vitamins and antioxidants.

- It can be used in soups, stews, curries, and mixed vegetable dishes.

- You can also use it raw to make juice or salad.

Avocado

Scientific Name: *Persea American*

Overview

Avocado, a fruit classified as a member of Lauraceae (a flowering plant family) is claimed to originate from south-central Mexico. It's a popular plant that is cultivated throughout the world in the Mediterranean and tropical climates.

Well known as butter fruit because of its creamy texture, avocado is a nutrient-dense fruit with a high amount of healthy monounsaturated fatty acids. It contains about 20 vitamins and minerals.

Health benefits

Nutrient-Dense: Avocado is a wonderful source of vitamins B-6, K, C, and E, folate, potassium, lutein, omega-3 fatty acid, riboflavin, pathogenic acid, niacin, magnesium, and beta-carotene.

Heart Health: a healthy cholesterol level is vital for the health of our heart. Beta-sitosterol plays a vital role in maintaining the cholesterol level

that is healthy for the heart.
Consuming plant sterols regularly
helps a lot and avocado contain
about 25mg/ounce of beta-
sitosterol.

Eye Health: Lutein and
zeaxanthin provided by avocado
serve as antioxidant protectors in
the eyes to reduce damage.

Osteoporosis: Vitamin K is very
vital for the bone. Vitamin K
helps to reduce the loss of
calcium through urinary excretion
and also facilitates calcium
absorption. Taking half if avocado

prices us with about 25% of the daily recommendation.

Cancer: although the true mechanism on how it works is yet to be known, researchers believe that the DNA and RNA are protected against undesirable mutations by folate during cell division. This folate helps to protect against cervical, stomach, colon, and pancreatic cancer.

Pregnancy: Folate also helps during pregnancy to reduce the risk of miscarriage and possible defects if the neural tube.

Depression: homocysteine impairs the delivery of nutrients to the brain. This substance also interferes with the production of dopamine, norepinephrine, and serotonin that controls sleep, appetite, and mood. Folate helps to prevent this homocysteine from building up.

Digestion: half of avocado contains 6-7 grams of fiber. Taking this with natural fiber helps to maintain the digestive tract and lower any risk of colon cancer.

Other health benefits of avocado include detoxification, antimicrobial action, protection and treatment of chronic disease and osteoporosis.

How To Use

It's important to know that we only use avocados in our meals when it ripens. How do you know when it's ripped? Gently press the skin. If it's soft and budge, then it's ripped. If not, give it some days to ripe.

You can use your avocados in your salads and sandwich, as

guacamole and dip. The avocado oil is used for cooking and also for moisturizing the skin.

CHAPTER 9

DR SEBI FOOD LIST

Vegetables

- ✓ Arame
- ✓ Wild Arugula
- ✓ Bell Pepper
- ✓ Zucchini
- ✓ Chayote
- ✓ Wakame
- ✓ Dulse
- ✓ Nopales
- ✓ Cucumber
- ✓ Garbanzo Beans
- ✓ Hijiki
- ✓ Sea Vegetables
- ✓ Avocado

- ✓ Dandelion Greens

- ✓ Izote flower and leaf

- ✓ Kale

- ✓ Cherry and Plum Tomato

- ✓ Mushrooms except Shitake

- ✓ Lettuce except iceberg

- ✓ Olives

- ✓ Nori

- ✓ Onions

- ✓ Purslane Verdolaga

- ✓ Squash

- ✓ Tomatillo

- ✓ Turnip Greens

- ✓ Amaranth

- ✓ Watercress
- ✓ Okra

Fruits

- ✓ Tamarind
- ✓ Prickly Pear
- ✓ Peaches
- ✓ Bananas
- ✓ Figs
- ✓ Prunes
- ✓ Cherries
- ✓ Berries
- ✓ Rasins
- ✓ Currants

- ✓ Pears
- ✓ Dates
- ✓ Orange
- ✓ Grapes
- ✓ Limes
- ✓ Mango
- ✓ Plums
- ✓ Apples
- ✓ Soft Jelly Coconuts
- ✓ Melons
- ✓ Cantaloupe
- ✓ Papayas
- ✓ Soursoups

Spices and Seasonings

✓ Sage

✓ Achiote

✓ Sweet Basil

✓ Basil

✓ Dill

✓ Habanero

✓ Cayenne

✓ Bay Leaf

✓ Onion Powder

✓ Oregano

✓ Pure Sea Salt

✓ Thyme

✓ Savory

- ✓ Cloves
- ✓ Tarragon
- ✓ Powdered Granulated Seaweed

Grains

- ✓ Fonio
- ✓ Spelt
- ✓ Kamut
- ✓ Rye
- ✓ Tef
- ✓ Amaranth
- ✓ Quinoa
- ✓ Wild Rice

Sugars and Sweeteners

- ✓ Sugar (gotten from dried dates)
- ✓ Agave Syrup gotten from cactus (100% Pure)

Herbal Teas

- ✓ Chamomile

- ✓ Red Raspberry

- ✓ Elderberry

- ✓ Fennel

- ✓ Burdock

- ✓ Ginger

- ✓ Tila

Nuts and Seeds

- ✓ Brazil Nuts

- ✓ Raw Sesame Seeds

- ✓ Hemp seeds

- ✓ Walnuts

Oils

- ✓ Avocado Oil

- ✓ Sesame Oil

- ✓ Coconut Oil

- ✓ Grapeseed Oil

- ✓ Hempseed Oil

- ✓ Olive Oil

OTHER BOOKS BY THE SAME AUTHOR

Dr. Sebi Mucus Cleanse

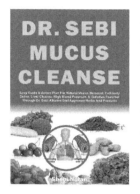

Link to kindle edition: https://www.amazon.co m/dp/B08G4Z3D8H

Link to print edition: https://www.amazon.co m/DR-SEBI-MUCUS-CLEANSE-Full-body/dp/B08GB253XW

Dr. Sebi Fasting For Weight Loss, Treatment And Cure

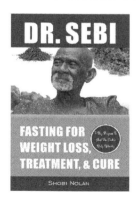

Link to kindle edition: https://www.amazon.co m/dp/B08H1HXCSN

Link to print edition: https://www.amazon.co m/SEBI-FASTING-WEIGHT-LOSS-TREATMENT/dp/B08G VGCDC2

Dr. Sebi Alkaline Diet Detox Guide For Women

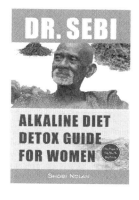

Link to kindle edition: https://www.amazon.com/dp/B08H2FSSJ5

Link to print edition: https://www.amazon.com/SEBI-ALKALINE-DETOX-GUIDE-WOMEN/dp/B08GVGD18H

Dr. Sebi Natural Blood Pressure Control

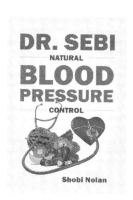

Link to kindle edition: https://www.amazon.com/dp/B08JCKFNNL

Link to print edition: https://www.amazon.com/SEBI-NATURAL-BLOOD-PRESSURE-CONTROL/dp/B08JB1XH13

Dr. Sebi Approved 3-Day Mucus Buster Diet For Women

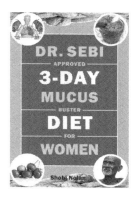

Link to kindle edition: https://www.amazon.com/dp/B08GMBD8DX

Link to print edition: https://www.amazon.com/APPROVED-3-DAY-MUCUS-BUSTER-WOMEN/dp/B08GVJTRNY

Dr Sebi 7-Day Cure For Herpes

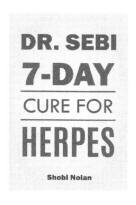

Link to kindle edition: https://www.amazon.com/dp/B08KGYVP8M

Dr Sebi Easy Guide To Stop Drinking Alcohol

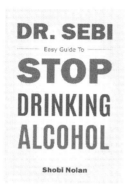

Link to kindle edition: https://www.amazon.com/dp/B08KH2L5RZ

Dr Sebi Low Cholesterol Diet

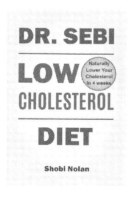

Link to kindle edition: https://www.amazon.com/dp/B08KGZZKBP

Dr Sebi Easy Way To Stop Smoking

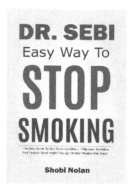

Link to kindle edition:
https://www.amazon.co
m/dp/B08J9QNZBR

Link to print edition:
https://www.amazon.co
m/SEBI-EASY-WAY-
STOP-
SMOKING/dp/B08JF5C
ZBZ

Dr. Sebi Diet Guide To Stop Acid Reflux

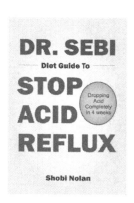

Link to kindle edition:
https://www.amazon.co
m/dp/B08JB29WD8

Link to print edition:
https://www.amazon.co
m/SEBI-DIET-GUIDE-
STOP-
REFLUX/dp/B08JF29R
HF

The New Breath - Dr. Sebi's Natural Science To Stop Asthma

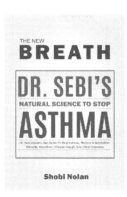

Link to kindle edition: https://www.amazon.com/dp/B08JB565XR

Link to print edition: https://www.amazon.com/NEW-BREATH-Inflammation-Sinusitis-Heartburn/dp/B08JF5CS15

Dr. Sebi Alkaline Herbal Cure In 28 days

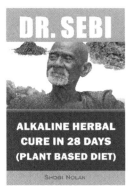

Link to kindle edition: https://www.amazon.com/dp/B08H1G3CQQ

Link to print edition: https://www.amazon.com/Sebi-Alkaline-Herbal-PLANT-BASED/dp/B08GVLWJVJ

The Dr. Sebi Diabetes Cure Book

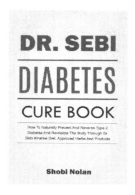

Made in the USA
Columbia, SC
10 May 2024

35541915R00109